The Mediterranean Vegetables Cookbook

A Complete Set of Vegetable-Based Mediterranean Recipes

Alex Brawn

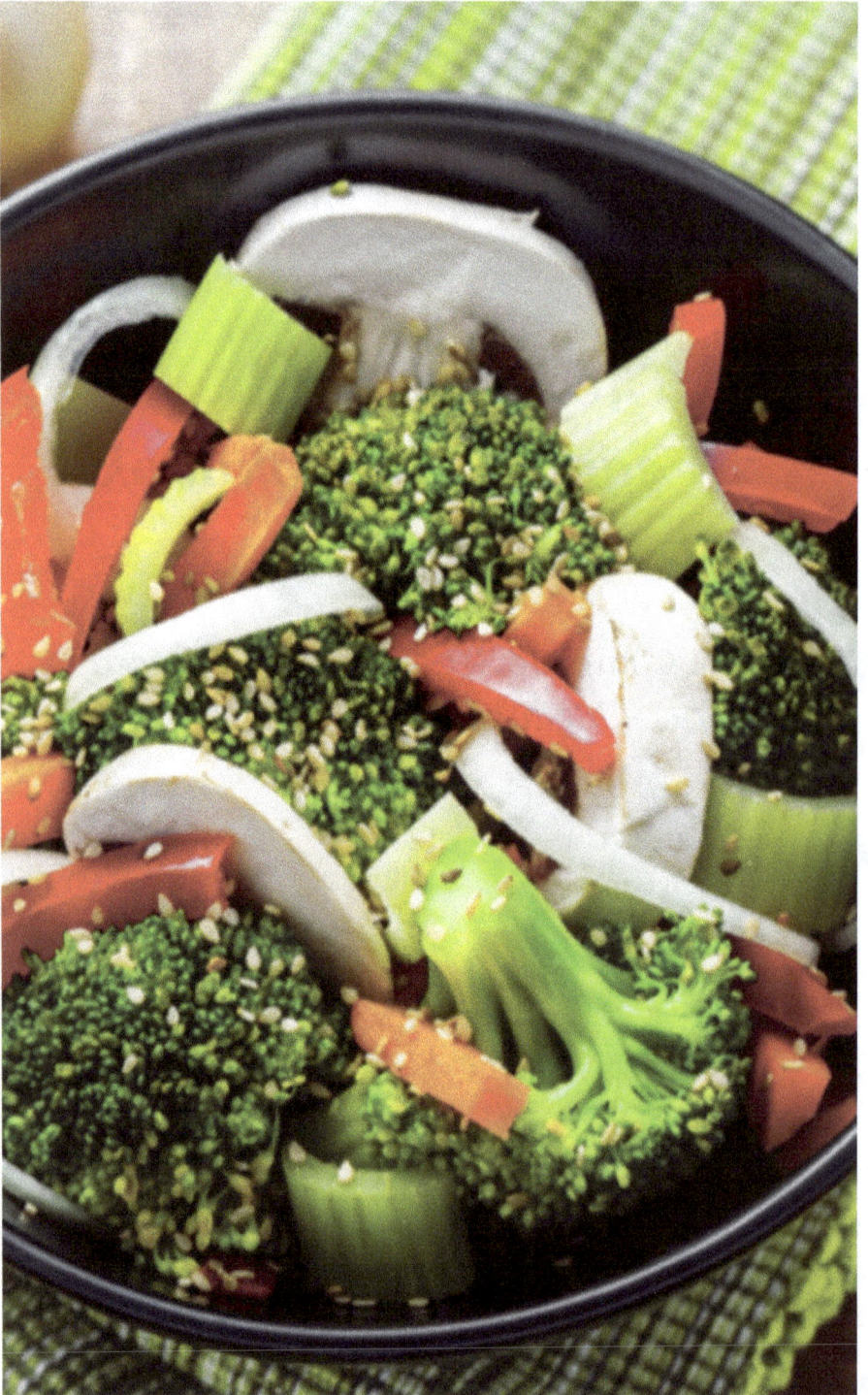

Table of Contents

Crispy Moroccan carrots

Ingredients

- 6 tablespoons of natural yoghurt
- 12 baby carrots
- Runny honey
- 3 oranges
- 2 teaspoons of rose harissa
- 1 tablespoon of tahini
- 3 fresh bay leaves
- 2 tablespoons of sesame seeds
- 3 sprigs of fresh thyme
- 4 sheets of filo pastry
- Olive oil

Directions

- Preheat the oven ready to 400°F.
- Place and cook the carrots in a pan of fast-boiling salted water for 10 minutes.
- Drain any excess water.
- Grate half the orange zest into the empty pan with all the juice.
- Place on a medium heat.

- Add the bay with thyme and a pinch of sea salt, let cook until syrupy.
- Fold carrots back into the glaze to coat. Let cool.
- Lay out the filo sheets rubbed with oil, then cut lengthways into 3 strips.
- Place a carrot at the bottom of each and roll up.
- Repeat for all the carrots and filo.
- Transfer to a baking tray.
- Brush each lightly with oil, let roast for 20 minutes.
- Drizzle with a little honey and scattering with the sesame seeds for last 5 minutes.
- Stack the carrots on a board, swirl the tahini and harissa through the yoghurt.
- Serve and enjoy.

Rogan josh scotch eggs

Ingredients

- mango chutney
- 5 large free-range eggs
- 2 liters of vegetable oil
- 2 x 250 g packets of mixed cooked grains
- 50g of plain flour
- 2 heaped teaspoons of Rogan josh curry paste
- 1 bunch of fresh mint
- 1 naan bread

Directions

- Start by soft-boiling 4 eggs in a pan of boiling salted water on a medium heat for 5 minutes.
- Drain, let cool under running water. Peel.
- Place the grains into a food processor with the curry paste, mint leaves, process until tacky in texture.
- Divide into 4 balls.
- Pat one at a time on a greaseproof paper.

- Place the paper flat on your hand, put a peeled egg in the center and mold the mixture up and around the egg to seal it inside.
- Remove the ball from the paper, press in hands to create the perfect covering.
- Place the flour in one bowl, beat the remaining egg in a separate bowl, add the naan to fine crumbs into a third bowl.
- Cover the coated eggs with flour, dip into the beaten egg and roll in the crumbs.
- Place on a medium-high heat.
- Lower the Scotch eggs into the pan let cook for 8 minutes.
- Scoop out and drain on kitchen paper.
- Serve and enjoy.

Moroccan salad with blood oranges, olives, almond and mint

Ingredients

- 1 teaspoon of honey , maple
- 1 ¾ cups of water
- Pinch of salt
- 12 fresh mint leaves, torn
- 2 green onions, sliced diagonally
- 1 tablespoon of red wine vinegar
- 1 cup of rinsed quinoa
- ¼ cup of thinly sliced Kalamata olives
- cracked pepper and salt to taste
- ¼ cup of toasted slivered
- 3 blood oranges- divided
- ¼ cup of olive oil

Directions

- Boil quinoa in salted water in a medium pot on the stove.
- Lower heat once boiling, cover and cook for15 minutes.

- In a medium bowl, add sliced green onions with sliced olives, and 2 oranges.
- Toss the quinoa in the bowl with the oranges.
- Dress with 4 tablespoons of olive oil , zest and juice of the remaining orange, and honey . Stir.
- Taste and adjust accordingly.
- Scatter with toasted slivered almonds and fresh torn mint leaves.
- Serve and enjoy warm or chilled.

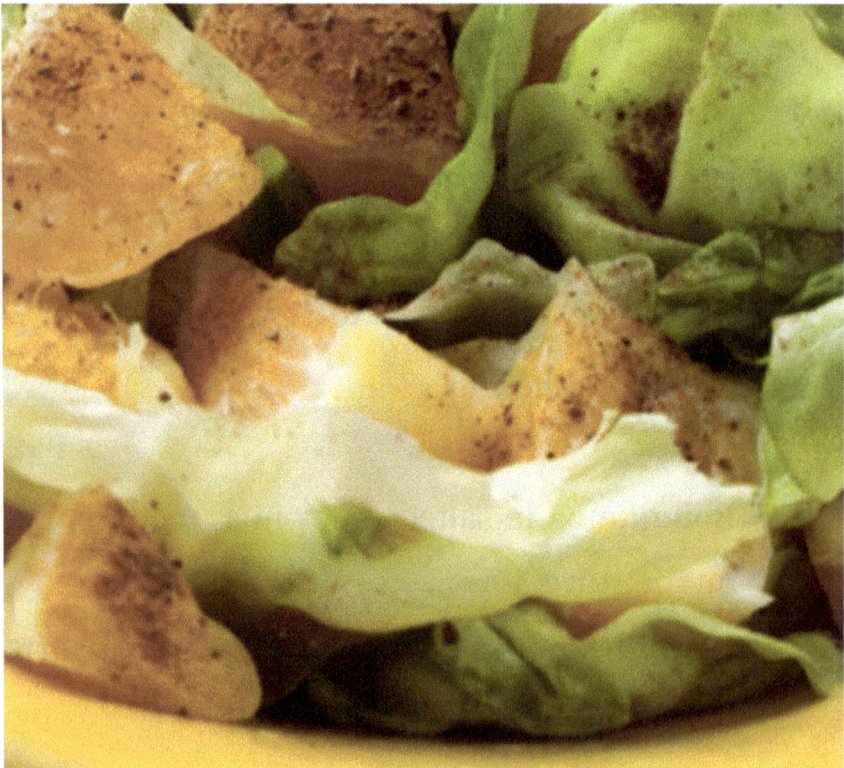

Warm grape and radicchio salad

The warm grape and radicchio salad recipe is carefully charred under the grill with incredible fresh balsamic and honey for a sweeter taste.

Ingredients

- 30g of rocket
- 200g of seedless red grapes
- 1 radicchio or 2 red chicory
- 1 tablespoon of runny honey
- 2 tablespoons of balsamic vinegar
- Olive oil
- 2 cloves of garlic
- 2 sprigs of fresh rosemary
- 2 heaped tablespoons of pine nuts

Directions

- Place grapes on a griddle pan over a high heat let grill for 5 minutes.
- Transfer in a large salad bowl.
- Working in batches, grill, char the radicchio to soften on both sides.
- Add to the bowl.

- Add garlic, rosemary leaves, pine nuts, and oil in the still-hot griddle pan.
- Add the balsamic vinegar together with the honey. Toss.
- Seasoning with sea salt and black pepper.
- Let settle for 10 minutes, then toss.
- Serve and enjoy.

Nordic nicoise salad

Ingredients

- 2 teaspoons of fresh grated
- 1 tablespoon of chopped fresh dill
- 2 eggs
- 1 cup of snap peas
- 1 cucumber
- Pinch sugar
- 1 tablespoon of finely chopped shallot
- 4 radishes
- 6 ounces of smoked trout
- 1 tablespoon of capers
- 2 tablespoons of fresh dill
- ¼ cup of olive oil
- 2 tablespoons of champagne vinegar
- 8 baby potatoes
- 1 teaspoon of wholegrain mustard
- 1 bunch watercress
- ¼ teaspoon of salt
- ¼ teaspoon of white pepper

Directions

- Boil potatoes, let simmer until tender in 20 minutes.
- Add the snap peas in the same water during the last minute.
- Drain. Rinse under cold water.
- Boil the eggs.
- Stir in olive oil, champagne vinegar, mustard, shallot, dill, salt, sugar, white pepper, and horseradish, tasting and adjust.
- Serve and enjoy with the vegetables salad.

Roasted black bean burgers

The roasted black bean burger features variety of fruits and vegetables typically mango, avocado, tabasco, tomatoes among others, making a perfect Mediterranean Sea diet.

Ingredients

- 1 ripe avocado
- 1½ red onions
- 200g of mixed mushrooms
- Chipotle tabasco sauce
- 4 tablespoons of natural yoghurt
- 100g of rye bread
- Ground coriander
- 1 x 400 g tin of black beans
- 4 sprigs of fresh coriander
- Olive oil
- 40g of mature cheddar cheese
- 1 ripe mango
- 4 soft rolls
- 100g of ripe cherry tomatoes
- 1 lime

Directions

- Preheat the oven ready to 400°F.
- Place 1 onion in a food processor with rye bread mushrooms, and ground coriander process until fine.
- Drain, pulse in the black beans
- Season lightly with sea salt and black pepper.
- Divide into 4 and shape into patties.
- Rub with oil and dust with ground coriander.
- Transfer to oiled baking tray let roast for 25 minutes, until dark and crispy.
- Top with the Cheddar, then warm the rolls.
- Combine the onions and tomatoes in a bowl.
- Squeeze over the lime juice with a bit of Tabasco.
- Season to taste.
- Halve the warm rolls and divide the yoghurt between the bases, and half of the salsa, avocado, mango, and coriander leaves.
- Top with the burgers and the balance of salsa and press down lightly.
- Serve and enjoy.

Brilliant bhaji burger

Ingredients

- 2 fresh green chilies
- 75g of paneer cheese
- 200g of butternut squash
- Mango chutney
- 4cm piece of ginger
- 100g of plain flour
- 1 lime
- 2 teaspoons of Rogan josh curry paste
- 2 cloves of garlic
- 2 uncooked poppadum
- Olive oil
- 4 soft burger buns
- 1 red onion
- 1 big bunch of fresh coriander
- 75g of natural yoghurt
- 1 baby gem lettuce

Directions

- Combine onion, garlic, chilies, and coriander stalks in a bowl.

- Add paneer with squash, ginger.
- Sprinkle in the flour and a pinch of sea salt and black pepper.
- Squeeze over the lime juice.
- Add the curry paste and water, mix.
- Drizzle 2 tablespoons of oil into a large non-stick frying pan over a medium heat.
- Divide the mixture into 4 portions and place in the pan.
- Let fry for 16 minutes, turning every few minutes.
- Then pound most of the coriander leaves to a paste in a pestle, muddle in the yoghurt, season.
- Divide the coriander yoghurt between the bases and inside bun-lids, then break up the poppadoms and sprinkle over.
- Place a crispy bhaji burger on top of each bun-base.
- Add a dollop of mango chutney, coriander leaves, and the lettuce.
- Serve and enjoy chilled.

Summer Tagliatelle

Ingredients

- 1 potato
- ½ a clove of garlic
- 200g of delicate summer vegetables
- 50g of blanched almonds
- 300g of Tagliatelle
- Extra virgin olive oil
- 25g of Parmesan cheese
- ¼ of a lemon
- 1 bunch of fresh basil
- 125g of green beans

Directions

- Place most of the basil leaves into a pestle pulse to a paste with a pinch of sea salt.
- Add in the garlic with pounded almonds until fine.
- Muddle in 4 tablespoons of oil with parmesan, squeeze of lemon juice.
- Season accordingly.

- Place sliced potatoes and beans in a pan of boiling salted water with Tagliatelle.
- Let cook as per the pasta packet Directions.
- Add delicate summer vegetables to the pan for the last 3 minutes.
- Drain, and keep some cooking water, then toss with the pesto, loosening with a splash of reserved water.
- Drizzle with 1 tablespoon of oil, complete with basil.
- Serve and enjoy with crunchy salad.

Roasted tomato risotto

Ingredients

- 450g of Arborio risotto rice
- 80g of Parmesan cheese
- 1 bulb of fennel
- 1 bulb of garlic
- ½ a bunch of fresh thyme
- 150ml of dry white vermouth
- Olive oil
- 1.2 liters of organic vegetable stock
- 1 onion
- 2 knobs of unsalted butter
- 6 large ripe tomatoes

Directions

- Preheat the oven ready to 350°F.
- Remove tomatoes seeds, place in a snug-fitting baking dish with cut sides up with garlic bulb.
- Spread with thyme sprigs.
- Drizzle with 1 tablespoon of oil.
- Season with sea salt, let roast until starting to burst open.

- Bring the stock to a simmer.
- Place onions with olive oil and knob of butter in a large pan on a medium heat. butter.
- Cook until softened, stirring occasionally.
- Stir in the rice, toast for 2 minutes.
- Pour in the vermouth, stir until absorbed.
- Add the stock let it be fully absorbed, then add another, stirring constantly until the rice is cooked in 18 minutes.
- Beat in the remaining knob of butter, Parmesan.
- Season and turn off the heat.
- Let rest for 2 minutes.
- Divide the risotto between warm plates, place a tomato in the center with sweet garlic and the herby fennel.
- Serve and enjoy.

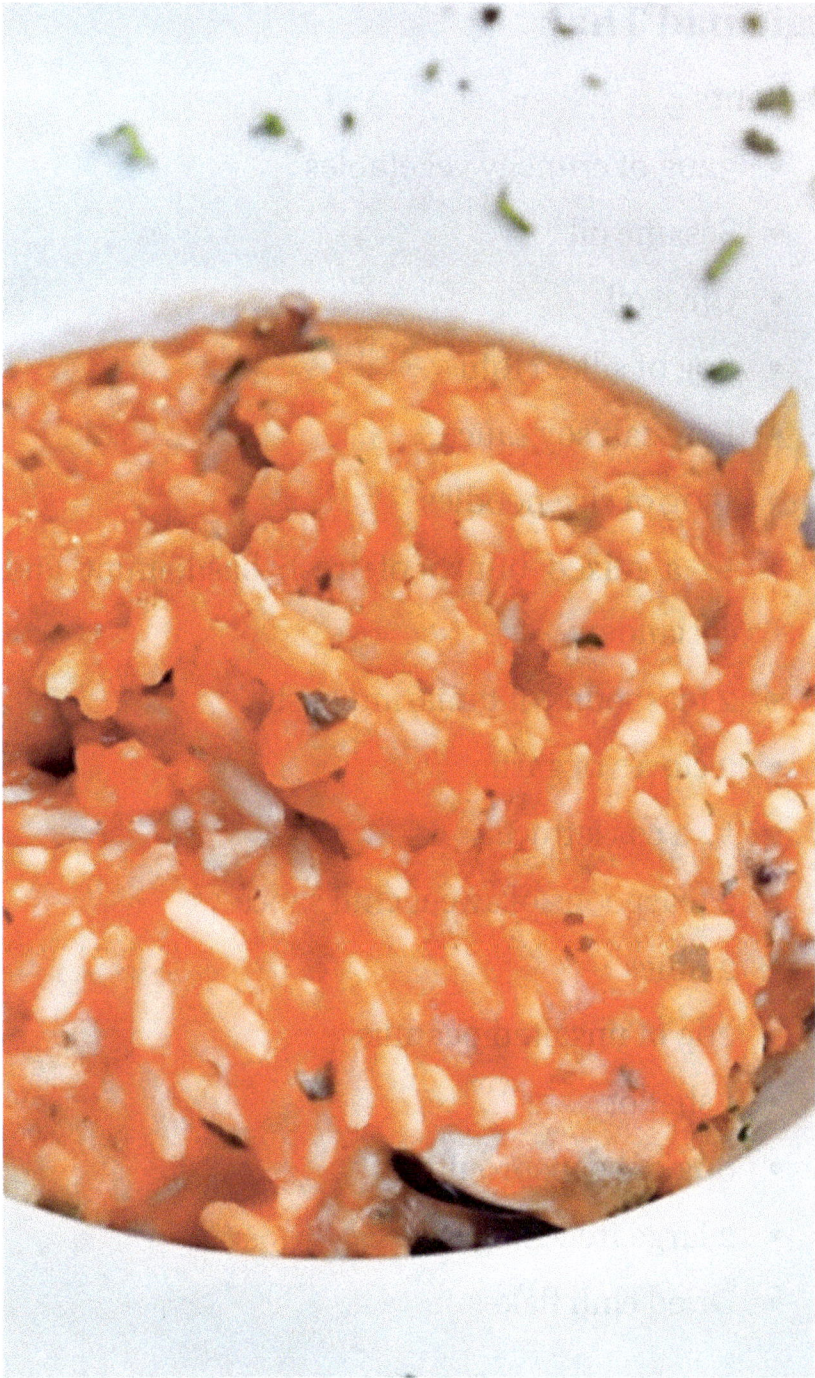

Veggie pad Thai

Ingredients

- 320g of crunchy vegetables
- Sesame oil
- Olive oil
- 80g of silken tofu
- Low-salt soy sauce
- 150g of rice noodles
- ½ a mixed bunch of fresh basil, mint and coriander
- 2 teaspoons of tamarind paste
- 2 cloves of garlic
- ½ a cos lettuce
- 2 teaspoons of sweet chili sauce
- 2 limes
- 20g of unsalted peanuts
- 1 shallot
- 80g of beansprouts
- 2 large free-range eggs
- Dried chili flakes

Directions

- Start by cook the noodles according to the packet Directions.
- Drain any excess water, toss with 1 teaspoon of sesame oil.
- Toast the peanuts in a large non-stick frying pan on a medium heat until golden.
- Blend in a pestle until fine, place into a bowl.
- Bash the garlic to a paste with the tofu.
- Add sesame oil with soy, tamarind paste, and chili sauce.
- Muddle in half the lime juice.
- Place slices of shallot in a frying pan over a high heat.
- Dry-fry the crunchy veggies for 4 minutes.
- Add the noodles together with sauce, beansprouts, and splash of water, toss over heat for 1 minute.
- Wipe out the pan, crack in the eggs let cook in a little olive oil, sprinkled with a pinch of chili flakes.

- Place lettuce in the bowls with eggs on top and pick over the herbs.
- Serve and enjoy with lime wedges.

Pea and ricotta stuffed courgettes

Ingredients

- 2 cloves of garlic
- 4 sprigs of fresh mint
- olive oil
- 100g of ricotta cheese
- 50g of mature Cheddar cheese
- 300g of basmati rice
- 1 lemon
- 8 baby courgettes, with flowers
- 400g of ripe cherry tomatoes
- red wine vinegar
- 150g of fresh or frozen peas
- 4 spring onions
- 8 black olives
- 1 fresh red chili

Directions

- Preheat the oven ready to 400°F.
- Process the mint leaves in a food processor with peas, ricotta, and Cheddar.

- Squeeze in the lemon juice with black pepper, blend until smooth.
- Taste and adjust the seasoning.
- Fill each courgette flower with the mixture, seal the petals.
- Place the tomatoes, onions, and olives roasting tray.
- Drizzle with 2 tablespoons each of oil and vinegar, season with pepper.
- Stir in the rice and boiling water, bring to the boil, stirring occasionally.
- Bake the courgettes inside rice for 20 minutes until golden.
- Serve and enjoy with summery salad

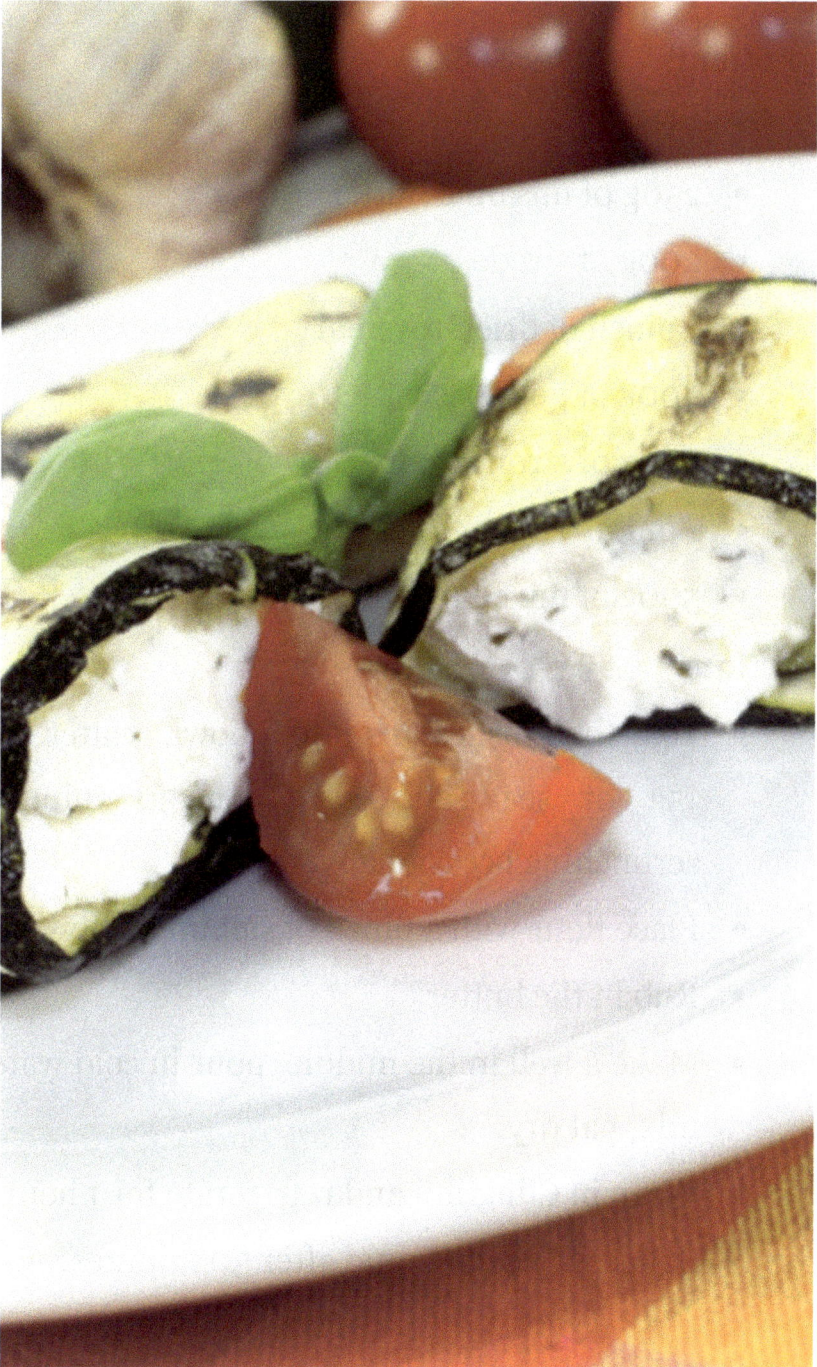

Veggie pasties

Ingredients

- 1 large free-range egg
- 250g of unsalted butter
- 200g of swede
- 1 pinch of dried rosemary
- 400g of potatoes
- 500g of strong flour
- 1 onion
- 500g of mixed mushrooms

Directions

- Tear the mushrooms into a bowl, scatter over 15g of sea salt, leave for 30 minutes, scrunching occasionally.
- Place flour with a pinch of salt into a bowl.
- Rub in the butter.
- Make a well in the middle, pour in cold water, mix, pat dry.
- Wrap in Clingfilm and refrigerate for 1 hour.
- Squeeze to salty liquid after 30 minutes.

- Mix the veggies with the mushrooms, rosemary and pinches of black pepper.
- Preheat the oven to 350°F.
- Divide the pastry into 8, then roll out into rounds.
- Divide up the filling, then scrunch and pile it to one side of the middle.
- Brush the exposed pastry with beaten egg, fold over and press the edges down, seal with your thumb. Egg wash.
- Place on a lined baking sheet let bake for 40 minutes.
- Serve and enjoy with watercress.

Asparagus quiche and soup

Ingredients

- 1.5 liters of organic vegetable stock
- 125g of whole meal flour
- 2 onions
- 150g of mature Cheddar cheese
- 125g of unsalted butter
- 7 large free-range eggs
- 1kg of asparagus
- 150g of ricotta cheese
- Olive oil
- 125g of plain flour
- 2 large potatoes
- ½ a bunch of fresh thyme

Directions

- Preheat the oven to 350°F.
- Put flours into a bowl with pinch of sea salt, rub in the butter.
- Make a well in the middle, crack in one of the eggs, mix with cold water, pat dry and bring together.

- Place between two large sheets of greaseproof paper, flatten, chill for 30 minutes.
- Roll out the pastry between the sheets, line a loose-bottomed tart tin with the pastry, bake for 20 minutes.
- Place asparagus and oil in a large pan over a medium heat.
- Add the potatoes with onions, thyme leaves cook until lightly golden, stirring regularly.
- Pour in the stock, boil, then simmer for 15 minutes.
- Blend until smooth, sieve.
- Season to taste with salt and black pepper.
- Beat the remaining eggs in a bowl with a pinch of salt and pepper.
- Add the ricotta with Cheddar and remaining thyme leaves.
- Stir the asparagus into the egg mixture and tip into the tart case.
- Let bake for 40 minutes.
- Serve and enjoy.

Summer vegetable blanket pie

Ingredients

- 320g of ripe cherry tomatoes
- 4 cloves of garlic
- 1 tablespoon of fennel seeds
- Olive oil
- 1 pinch of saffron
- 320g of potatoes
- 320g of butternut squash
- 320g of courgettes
- 1 tablespoon of sesame seeds
- ½ x 700g jar of chickpeas
- 1 large leek
- Extra virgin olive oil
- 8 sheets of filo pastry
- 1 preserved lemon
- 1 tablespoon of red wine vinegar
- 400g of natural yoghurt
- 1 teaspoon of rose harissa
- 50g of dried sour cherries

Directions

- Sieve the yogurt through into a bowl, then leave to drain.
- Season the tomatoes with sea salt and black pepper.
- Drizzle with extra virgin olive oil and the vinegar, then toss, let macerate.
- Preheat the oven to 375°F.
- Place garlic slices in a large frying pan on a medium heat with the fennel seeds and olive oil.
- Fry briefly, stirring regularly.
- Add potatoes, leek, and courgette let cook covered for 15 minutes.
- Add the chickpeas, season with a pinch of salt and pepper.
- Add lemon to the pan with a drizzle of juice from the jar, and the harissa.
- Continue to fry for 15 more minutes, stirring occasionally.

- Cover the sour cherries and saffron with boiling water, add tomatoes, reserving the macerating juices.
- Lay the filo out flat, then brush with tomato juices.
- Scatter over the sesame seeds and bake for 25 minutes
- Serve and enjoy with the pie.

Allotment cottage pie

The delicious taste of the allotment cottage pie will surprise anyone's taste buds. It is fully packed with variety of nutrients and a perfect Mediterranean Sea diet choice.

Ingredients

- 1 teaspoon of Marmite
- 2 large leeks
- 3 carrots
- 1 x 400g tin of green lentils
- 1 splash of semi-skimmed milk
- 10g of dried porcini mushrooms
- 500g of swede
- 500g of celeriac
- Olive oil
- 3 sprigs of fresh rosemary
- 1 onion
- 3 tablespoons of tomato purée
- 1 teaspoon cumin seeds
- 2kg of potatoes
- 40g of unsalted butter

Directions

- In a blender, cover the porcini with hot water.
- Drizzle oil into a large casserole pan over a medium heat.
- Fry the rosemary for 1 minute to crisp up.
- Add the cumin seeds together with prepared veggies to flavored oil.
- Season with sea salt and black pepper, cook for 30 minutes, stirring regularly.
- Cook the potatoes in a pan of boiling salted water until tender.
- Drain and mash with butter and milk, then season.
- Preheat the oven to 375°F.
- Add onions, marmite, tomato puree, blend until smooth.
- Pour into the veggie pan and cook for 20 minutes, stirring regularly.
- Place the lentils into the veg pan, boil, season to taste.
- Spoon over the mash, place on a tray.

- Let bake for 30 minutes, or until bubbling at the edges.
- Sprinkle over the crispy rosemary.
- Serve and enjoy with seasonal greens.

Sticky onion tart

The stick onion tart is quite flavorful with garlic and the onion itself. Above and beyond, this recipe is easy to make.

Ingredients

- 4 tablespoons of cider vinegar
- 4 medium onions
- 320g of sheet of all-butter puff pastry
- 50g of unsalted butter
- 8 cloves of garlic
- 4 sprigs of fresh thyme
- 4 fresh bay leaves
- 2 tablespoons of soft dark brown sugar

Directions

- Preheat the oven ready to 425°F.
- Place butter in an ovenproof frying pan on a medium heat.
- Add thyme leaves with the bay, sugar, vinegar, and water.
- Place the onion halves in the pan, cut side down with garlic in between.
- Season with sea salt and black pepper.

- Cover, over low heat and steam for 10 minutes to soften the onions, uncover cook until liquid starts to caramelize.
- Place the pastry over the onions, placed to the edge of the pan.
- Let bake for 35 minutes, until golden brown.
- Serve and enjoy.

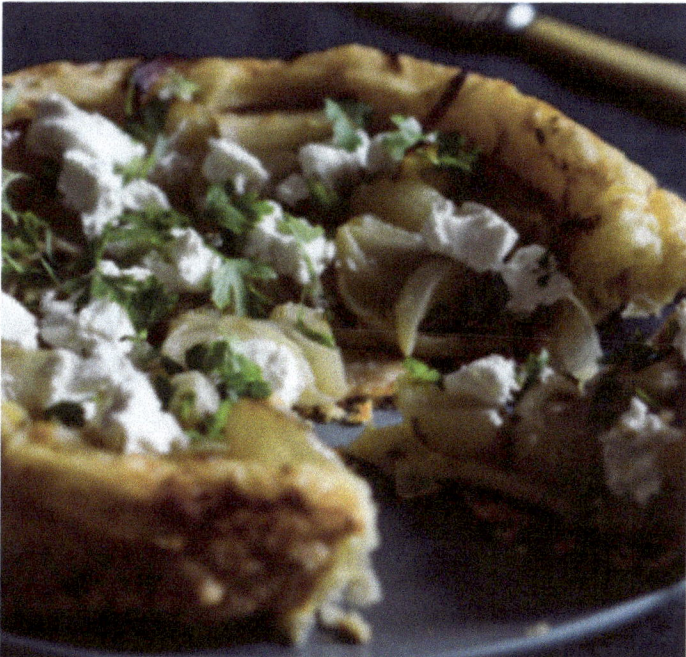

Tomato curry

Ingredients

- 2 teaspoons of mango chutney
- 1 onion
- 1.2kg of ripe mixed tomatoes
- 1 pinch of saffron
- 1 teaspoon of mustard seeds
- 1 teaspoon of fenugreek seeds
- 1 x 400g tin of light coconut milk
- 20g of flaked almonds
- 4 cloves of garlic
- 1 teaspoon of cumin seeds
- 4cm piece of ginger
- 2 fresh red chilies
- Olive oil
- 1 handful of fresh curry leaves

Directions

- Prick the tomatoes, plunge into fast-boiling water briefly.
- Peel the skin.

- Cover the saffron with boiling water and leave to infuse.
- Toast the almonds in a large non-stick frying pan over a medium heat until golden.
- Transfer to a small bowl and place the pan back on the heat.
- Drizzle 1 tablespoon of oil into the pan, add curry leaves with all the spices.
- Add onions with garlic, ginger, and chili to the pan, let fry for 3 minutes, stirring constantly.
- Add the tomatoes with the coconut milk and saffron water, let simmer for 20 minutes covered.
- Add mango chutney halfway.
- Season to taste with sea salt and black pepper, scatter over the almonds.
- Serve and enjoy with fluffy rice.

Vegetable chili

Ingredients

- 2 sweet potatoes
- 1 x 400g tin of cannellini beans
- 3 mixed-color peppers
- 4 large ripe tomatoes
- 1 lemon
- 1 bunch of fresh mint
- 4 tablespoons of natural yoghurt
- Olive oil
- 1 teaspoon of cumin seeds
- 1 teaspoon of smoked paprika
- 2 red onions
- 4 small flour tortillas
- 4 cloves of garlic
- Hot chili sauce
- 250g of black rice

Directions

- Preheat a griddle pan ready to high temperature.

- Drizzle 1 tablespoon of oil into a large casserole pan over a medium-low heat.
- Stir in the cumin with paprika, garlic, lemon zest, and grilled vegetables, stirring regularly.
- Add the beans and water, add chili sauce.
- Season with sea salt and black pepper let simmer for 30 minutes.
- Cook the rice in a pan of boiling salted water according to the packet Directions.
- Pick 2 sprigs of mint leaves and chop with the salsa veggie, toss with the lemon juice.
- Season to taste with salt and pepper.
- Warm the tortillas on the griddle and ripple shakes of chili sauce through the yoghurt.
- Serve and enjoy with black ricc.

Chicken and vegetable stir-fry

Ingredients

- 2 carrots
- ½ of a red onion
- 1 red pepper
- 80g of purple sprouting broccoli
- 1 tablespoon of reduced-salt soy sauce
- 80g of mixed mushrooms
- 1 free-range chicken breast
- 1 teaspoon of sesame seeds
- 1 tablespoon of sesame oil
- 4cm of piece of ginger
- 1 teaspoon of Chinese five-spice
- 1 teaspoon of vegetable oil
- Sprigs of fresh coriander
- 1 fresh red chili
- 1 clove of garlic
- 130g of baby corn
- 80g of mange tout
- 2 whole wheat noodle nests
- 1 tablespoon of black bean sauce

Directions

- Place the chicken into a bowl with the Chinese five-spice and sesame oil, toss.
- Place a large non-stick frying pan over a medium-high heat with the vegetable oil.
- Add the garlic together with the ginger and chili, toss briefly.
- Add the chicken let stir-fry for 2 minutes until golden.
- Add all the vegetables, let stir-fry for more 4 minutes.
- Cook the noodles as instructed on the package in a large pan of boiling salted water.
- Transfer the noodles to the pan, add soy with black bean sauce, toss to coat.
- Scatter over the sesame seeds and coriander.
- Serve and enjoy.

Roasted vegetable roots

Much as there are various ways one can roast veggies, the Mediterranean style is mega for a delicious and aromatic flavor with garlic taking the lead.

Ingredients

- 12 parsnips
- 3kg of potatoes
- 16 carrots
- ½ a bunch of fresh rosemary
- 1 bulb of garlic

Directions

- Begin by preheat your oven ready to 375°F.
- Cook potatoes with parsnips and carrots in a large pan of boiling salted water for 8 minutes.
- Drain any excess water in a colander let steam dry.
- Remove the carrots and parsnips put to one side, shakes the colander.
- Add 4 tablespoons of olive oil to two large roasting trays.
- Season each with sea salt and black pepper.

- Squash the garlic bulb, divide between the trays with the rosemary sprigs.
- Place in the veggies, red wine vinegar, toss to coat.
- Let roast for 40 minutes.
- Remove and squash with a fish slice to burst the skins.
- Place back in the oven for 20 minutes.
- Serve and enjoy.

Beetroot curry

What a blessing to add onto your body blood. Beet root is a gift to replenish blood in the body; as such, this recipe cannot be underestimated among Mediterranean Sea diets with earthly flavors.

Ingredients

- 1 teaspoon of hot curry powder
- 3 cloves of garlic
- 2 tablespoons of desiccated coconut
- 3 cloves of garlic
- 5cm of piece of ginger
- vegetable oil
- 2 teaspoons of black mustard seeds
- 1 kg mixed beets
- 250g of ripe cherry tomatoes
- 7g of dried curry leaves
- ½ a bunch of fresh coriander
- 320g of wild rice
- 6 spring onions
- 14g of dried curry leaves
- 5cm of piece of ginger

- 1 x 400ml tin of light coconut milk
- 1 lemon
- 1 lime
- 2 fresh long red chilies

Directions

- Place a large pan over a medium heat.
- Add the curry leaves with the curry powder, mustard seeds, and coconut, let toast for 2 minute. Transfer to a food processor and blend well.
- Add spring onions to the food processor with garlic, ginger, and vegetable oil.
- Pulse to forms a paste.
- Place the pan back on the hob over a medium heat.
- Add the paste cook briefly, add beetroot.
- Lower heat and cook until sticky and gnarly, stirring often.
- Add the cherry tomatoes and cook for 5 minutes, then break them with the back of a spoon.
- Cook the rice as instructed on the packet.

- Stir in the coconut milk with a squeeze of lemon juice.
- Raise the heat let cook for 5 minutes.
- Season to taste.
- Place a frying pan over a medium heat with oil.
- Add all the temper ingredients let heat for 2 minutes.
- Turn off the heat, transfer into a bowl lined with kitchen paper.
- Serve the curry with the rice and temper and or coriander leaves scattered on top.
- Serve and enjoy.

Brick lane burger

Everyone likes to enjoy a delicious burger, isn't it? If yes, then this Mediterranean Sea diet recipe is a must try for you. It has great flavors derived from onions, garlic and ginger.

Ingredients

- 200g of butternut squash
- 2 cloves of garlic
- 2 fresh green chilies
- 100g of paneer cheese
- Mango chutney
- 1 big bunch of fresh coriander
- 150g of gram flour
- 6 burger buns
- 2 teaspoons of ground turmeric
- 3 poppadoms
- 2 baby gem lettuce
- 1 carrot
- 2 teaspoons of ground cumin
- 2 red onions
- 2 limes

- Olive oil
- 100ml of natural yoghurt
- 5cm of piece of ginger
- 1 fresh red chili

Directions

- Preheat the oven to 350°F.
- Place onions, carrots, paneer, garlic, ginger, and coriander into a large mixing bowl.
- Place flour together with the turmeric and cumin.
- Season with sea salt and black pepper, squeeze in the juice of 1 lime with water, mix with your hands.
- Divide into 6, then shape and squash into patties.
- Drizzle with bit of oil into a large non-stick frying pan over a medium heat.
- Let fry the patties for 3 minutes on each side or until golden.
- Remove to a baking tray for 10 minutes or until cooked.

- Pestle the remaining coriander leaves, setting aside a handful.
- Add a pinch of salt, then bash to a paste. Squeeze in the juice of lime, stir in the yoghurt.
- Spoon a little coriander yoghurt over the base and inside lid of each burger bun.
- Crumble the poppadoms, sprinkle over the yoghurt, then sit a patty on top of each base and spread with 1 tablespoon of mango chutney.
- Top with a handful of lettuce and the reserved coriander leaves.
- Sprinkle with red chili
- Serve and enjoy.

Summer vegetable lasagna

Ingredients

- Olive oil
- ½ x 30g tin of anchovies in oil
- 6 cloves of garlic
- 500g of fresh lasagne sheets
- 700g of asparagus
- 1 lemon
- Sprigs of fresh thyme
- 500g of frozen peas
- 300g of frozen broad beans
- Parmesan cheese
- 1 bunch of spring onions
- 1 big bunch of fresh mint
- 300ml of single cream
- 300m of organic vegetable stock
- 2 x 250g tubs of cottage cheese

Directions

- Preheat the grill to full temperature.
- Pour oil from the anchovy tin into a large frying pan over a high heat

- Add the spring onions and anchovies.
- Add crushed garlic, toss well.
- Add asparagus stems to the pan, keep tips for later.
- Season with sea salt and black pepper.
- Add a splash of boiling water, let cook for a few minutes, stirring occasionally.
- Add the peas together with the broad beans, mint, lemon zest, and the cream to the pan.
- Squash, then season with salt and pepper.
- Pour in the stock and bring to the boil.
- Stir in 1 tub of cottage cheese.
- Place a roasting tray over a medium heat.
- Cover the bottom of the tray with the vegetable mixture, then top with a layer of lasagna sheets, and Parmesan grating.
- Repeat the layers with the rest of the vegetable mixture and pasta, use lasagne sheets to finish.
- Mix the remaining tub of cottage cheese with splash of water.

- Toss the reserved asparagus with a drizzle of oil.
- Strip over the thyme leaves.
- Turn the heat under the tray up to high and cook until the lasagne starts to bubble, place under the grill on the middle shelf for 8 minutes.
- Serve and enjoy.

Gnarly cauliflower curry

Ingredients

- ½ x 400g tin of light coconut milk
- 1 medium cauliflower
- 2 heaped tablespoons of rogan josh curry paste
- Extra virgin olive oil
- 2 heaped tablespoons of natural yoghurt
- 1 red onion
- 1 pinch of dried red chili flakes
- 2 cloves of garlic
- 150g of basmati rice
- 2 lemons
- 4 uncooked poppadoms
- ½ a bunch of fresh coriander
- Pickled chilies

Directions

- Preheat the grill to high.
- Place prepared cauliflower in a large pan.
- Rub the cauliflower with Rogan josh paste.
- Season with sea salt and black pepper.

- Add in the cauliflower leaves then place over a medium heat on the hob with water.
- Add in the garlic, onions, on top of the cauliflower.
- Bring to the boil, let bubble for 10 minutes.
- Transfer the pan to the grill, 5cm away, for 15 minutes or until gnarly, charred and cooked through.
- Cook the rice in a pan of boiling salted water per the packet instruction with half a lemon, drain excess water.
- Pick the coriander leaves from 1 sprig and scatter over with a few pickled chilies and liquor. Mix.
- Drizzle with 1 tablespoon of oil.
- Remove the cauliflower, place over a medium heat.
- Pour in the coconut milk let boil, stirring gently.
- One-by-one, puff up your dry poppadoms in the microwave briefly.

- Add coriander stalks to a pestle with a pinch of salt and chili flakes blend to a paste.
- Muddle in the yoghurt.
- Sprinkle the coriander leaves over the curry, add lemon into rice.
- Serve and enjoy with poppadoms, and lemon pickle.

Pot roasted cauliflower

Ingredients

- 1 small pinch of saffron
- Olive oil
- 1 large head of cauliflower
- 6 cloves of garlic
- 3 onions
- 6 large green olives
- 6 anchovy fillets in oil
- 500ml of white wine

Directions

- Preheat the oven to 350°F.
- Combine onions, olive oil, and anchovies in an ovenproof pan on a medium-high heat.
- Add olive with the garlic let cook for 2 minutes, pour in the wine with saffron.
- Sit the cauliflower in the pan, stalk side down.
- Drizzle with 1 tablespoon of oil.
- Spoon bit of onions and liquid over the cauliflower, boil.
- Transfer the pan to the oven for 1 hour.

- Carefully lift the cauliflower on to a platter and spoon over the soft onions, olives and fragrant juices from the pan.
- Serve and enjoy with sliced onions and olives.

Peas, beans, chili and mint

Ingredients

- 1 lemon
- 1 fresh red chili
- 200g of fresh podded
- ½ a bunch of fresh mint
- 200g of fresh podded

Directions

- Put the mint stalks in a pan of boiling salted water, with the beans and peas to cook for 4 minutes.
- Combine leafy mint, lemon zest, extra virgin oil, and chili in a bowl, mix.
- Season with sea salt and black pepper.
- Drain the beans and peas, reserving some cooking water for later.
- Pinch the skins off any larger beans, pour the beans and peas on to a platter, toss with a few splashes of reserved cooking water, then spoon over the dressing.
- Drizzle with extra virgin olive oil and toss together.

- Serve and enjoy.

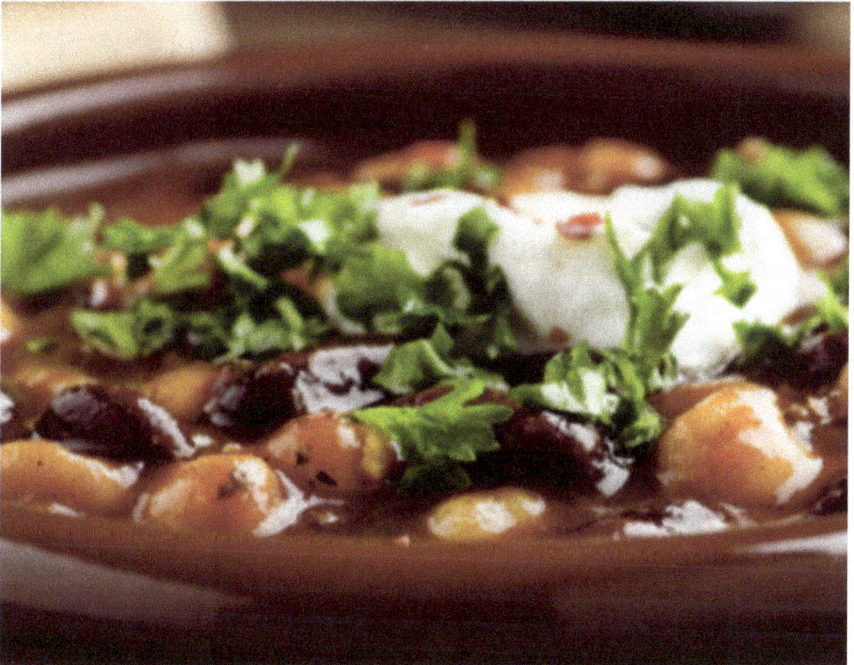

Dressed beets

This recipe embraces the healthy benefits of beets, citrus, vinegar and walnuts for a perfect Mediterranean Sea diet.

Ingredients

- 100g of crumbly goat's cheese
- 4 clementine
- 600g of raw mixed-color baby beets
- 40g of shelled unsalted walnut halves
- Extra virgin olive oil
- Red wine vinegar
- ½ a bunch of fresh tarragon

Directions

- Cook the beets covered, in a pan of boiling salted water for 20 minutes.
- Squeeze the juice of 1 clementine into a large bowl with extra virgin olive oil and red wine vinegar.
- Slice and arrange remaining clementine on a plates.
- Drain the beets rub off the skins when cooled under running water.

- Season with sea salt and black pepper, add the tarragon and toss with the reserved beet leaves.
- Divide between your plates, crumble over the goat's cheese and walnuts.
- Serve an enjoy drizzled with extra virgin olive oil.

Roasted roots halloumi tray bake with courgette tangles

Ingredients

- 4 tablespoons of quality green pesto
- 1 small broccoli
- Olive oil
- 800g of mixed root veggies
- 250g of halloumi cheese
- 2 red peppers
- 1 large eating apple
- 1 courgette
- 100g of lamb's lettuce

Directions

- Preheat the oven to 400°F.
- Spread the veg out on a large roasting tray.
- Drizzle with olive oil.
- Then, season with sea salt and black pepper, toss to coat.
- Let roast until the vegetables are tender and colored.
- Cut and scatter over the veggies.

- Switch the oven to grill, raise the heat and grill for 10 minutes.
- Spiralize the courgette.
- Combine sliced apple with the roasted veggies, then stir through the courgetti and spinach.
- Mix the pesto with 2 tablespoons of oil and drizzle over.
- Serve and enjoy.

Parsnip beetroot gratin

Ingredients

- 2 oranges
- 500g of beetroots
- 300ml of double cream
- Unsalted butter
- ½ a bunch of fresh rosemary
- 200ml of crème fraiche
- 500g of parsnips
- 4 cloves of garlic

Directions

- Preheat the oven to 400°F.
- Oil a 1.5-liter baking dish ready.
- Layer up sliced parsnips and beets in the baking dish.
- Put the cream together with the crème fraîche, whole unpeeled garlic, and rosemary sprigs in a saucepan, let simmer.
- Remove the heat, add orange zest.
- Season with sea salt and a big pinch of black pepper.

- Pour the cream over the vegetables, pressing them to submerge in the liquid and arrange the rosemary sprigs on top.
- Cover tightly with tin foil
- Let bake for 45 minutes, until the vegetable is almost tender.
- Remove the foil and continue to bake for 25 minutes.
- Cool for 5 minutes.
- Serve and enjoy.

Roasted radish and runner bean tray bake

Ingredients

- 25g of Cheddar cheese
- 1 tablespoon of red wine vinegar
- 150g of runner beans
- 70g of ciabatta
- Sprigs of fresh dill, flat-leaf parsley, chives
- 6 radishes, with tops
- 3 cloves of garlic
- 1 teaspoon of runny honey
- 100ml of white wine
- 2 courgettes
- Olive oil
- Extra virgin olive oil

Directions

- Preheat the oven to 375°F.
- Pour in the wine or stock.
- Season with sea salt and black pepper, drizzle over 2 tablespoons of olive oil.
- Coarsely blend the cheddar and sprinkle over the bread pieces.

- Let roast in the oven for 40 minutes or until cooked through.
- Combine 2 tablespoons of extra virgin olive oil with the honey and vinegar.
- Stir through the chopped herbs, season and keep aside.
- Remove the tray from the oven and drizzle with the dressing.
- Serve and enjoy on a bed of spinach.

Apricot, root veggie cake with honey yogurt icing

Ingredients

- 150g of Greek-style natural yoghurt
- 40g of pumpkin seeds
- 1 beetroot
- 2 parsnips
- 1 orange
- 1 lemon
- 120g of quality maple syrup
- 2 large free-range eggs
- 25g of clear runny honey
- 70 ml cold-pressed rapeseed oil
- 150g of wholegrain spelt flour
- 1 pinch of mixed spice
- 2 medium carrots
- 1 teaspoon baking powder
- 60g of dried apricots
- 150g of cream cheese
- ½ teaspoon of quality vanilla extract

Directions

- Preheat the oven to 350°F.
- Oil the base and sides of a loose-bottomed cake tin with a little rapeseed oil.
- Line the base with baking paper.
- Grate and combine the carrots, beetroot and parsnip into a large bowl.
- Add grated zest of the orange and 2/3 to the veggie with maple syrup, eggs, and rapeseed oil.
- Fold in the flour, spice, baking powder and a pinch of salt.
- Add diced apricot with seeds to the bowl, Mix to combine.
- Pour the mixture into the prepared tin lct bakc for 40 minutes, rotating the tin after 20 minutes.
- Let cool in the tin.
- Whisk together all the ingredients except the lemon, until smooth.
- Squeeze in a tiny bit of lemon juice and whisk again.

- Chill in the fridge until needed.
- Transfer to a plate finish with the icing.
- Slice and enjoy.

Roasted sprouts

Ingredients

- 1 small clove of garlic
- 500g of Brussels sprouts
- 1 lemon
- 25g of hazelnuts
- 2 teaspoons of coriander seeds
- 1 heaped teaspoon of tahini
- 2 small red onions
- ½ a bunch of fresh coriander
- 1 bulb of fennel
- Olive oil
- 1 pinch of sumac
- 1 teaspoon of sesame seeds
- 1 teaspoon of cumin seeds
- 200g of Greek yoghurt

Directions

- Preheat the oven to 400°F.
- Boil water salted in a large pan over a medium-high heat.
- Add sprouts to the pan let boil for 3 minutes.

- Drain excess water in a colander let dry.
- Toast the cumin together with the coriander seeds in a small frying pan over a medium heat until fragrant.
- Grind the toasted seeds with a pinch of sea salt using a mortar.
- Add the spice mix into a large roasting tray and toss with sprouts.
- Add onions into the tray with bit of oil.
- Spread everything in an even layer then, cook for 20 minutes.
- Return the frying pan to the heat and toast the sesame seeds together with the hazelnuts for 3 minutes.
- Grind up with the remaining spices, using a mortar.
- Combine the yoghurt with the tahini.
- Stir the crushed garlic through with lemon zest juice.
- Taste the yoghurt and season accordingly.
- Spread over the base of a large serving platter sprinkled with sumac.

- Spoon the sprout mix on top of the yoghurt mixture.
- Sprinkle the ground nuts and seeds over the top.
- Serve and enjoy with herb leaves scattered on the plate.

Whole roasted miso aubergine

Ingredients

- 1 tablespoon of tamarind paste
- 4 cloves of garlic
- 3 tablespoons of white sweet miso
- 2 small green chilies
- groundnut oil
- 200g of vine cherry tomatoes
- 3cm piece of ginger
- 4 spring onion
- ½ a bunch of coriander
- 1 lime
- 2 aubergines
- ½ tablespoon of honey

Directions

- Preheat your oven ready to 350°F.
- Grate the ginger into a large mortar and pestle, combine together with the garlic, chilies, and a pinch of salt, mix to form a thick paste.
- Spoon the mixture over the aubergines and massage it into the incisions on the meat.

- Place the aubergines in a large roasting tray.
- Dot the cherry tomatoes place into the oven for 40 minutes, turning occasionally.
- While the aubergines are cooking, trim and finely slice the spring onions and roughly chop the coriander, stalks and all. Add the onions together with the coriander stalks, squeeze over the lime juice to coat and mix well.
- Combine the tamarind with honey, miso, and water.
- Remove the roasting tray from the oven after 40 minutes.
- Raise the heat to high then drizzle the miso glaze over the aubergines.
- Return back into the oven for more 15 minutes.
- Remove the stalks from the aubergines and throw away.
- Chop the flesh in the tray into coarse chunks.
- Stir in the dressed spring onions.
- Serve and enjoy.

Roasted brassicas with puy lentil and halloumi

Ingredients

- 1 large bunch of mixed soft herbs
- Olive oil
- 1 heaped teaspoon of baharat
- 2 tablespoons of runny honey
- 4 cloves of garlic
- 250g of puy lentils
- 250g of halloumi cheese
- 1 liter of organic vegetable stock
- 800g of broccoli and cauliflower
- 1 fresh bay leaf
- 2 lemons
- Extra virgin olive oil
- 100g of walnuts

Direction

- Preheat the oven to 425°F.
- Spread out the broccoli and cauliflower in a single layer in a roasting tray.

- Drizzle with olive oil, then sprinkle with Baharat.
- Season with sea salt and black pepper.
- Toss in cloves of garlic, spread out in the tray.
- Roast for 25 minutes.
- Place lentils in a medium-sized pan.
- Pour over the hot stock, add the bay leaf.
- Boil over a medium heat, lower heat let simmer and cook for 30 minutes. Drain and set aside.
- Mash the garlic until creamy, add lemon juice let season and extra virgin olive oil. Season.
- Toast the walnuts with the herb leaves. Keep aside.
- Toss the hot lentils through the garlic dressing, with roasted veggies, herbs and nuts.
- Pour olive oil into a medium-sized, non-stick frying pan over a medium heat, fry the halloumi till golden.
- Drizzle with honey and fry for briefly.
- Serve and enjoy.

Lentil tabbouleh

Ingredients

- 1 lemon
- Extra virgin olive oil
- 1 bunch of spring onions
- 1 large bunch of fresh mint
- 200g of ripe cherry tomatoes
- 200g of lentils
- 1 large bunch of fresh flat-leaf parsley

Directions

- Cook the lentils in plenty of salted water until tender.
- Drain any excess water and set aside to cool.
- Mix the cooled lentils together with the tomatoes, spring onions, herbs, and 4 tablespoons of oil.
- Add the lemon juice.
- Season with sea salt and black pepper.
- Serve and enjoy.

Fresh mango salsa

The Mediterranean mango recipe is quite easy to make is few minutes. The colorful spicy salad is remarkable delicious especially when served with chips on tacos.

Ingredients

- 1 jalapeño, seeded and minced
- ¼ teaspoon salt, to taste
- 1 medium red bell pepper
- ½ cup of chopped red onion
- 3 ripe mangos
- 1 large lime, juiced
- ¼ cup of packed fresh cilantro leaves

Directions

- In a serving bowl, combine the prepared mango with bell pepper, onion, cilantro, and jalapeño.
- Drizzle with the juice of 1 lime.
- Stir the ingredients together.
- Season with salt.
- Serve an enjoy.

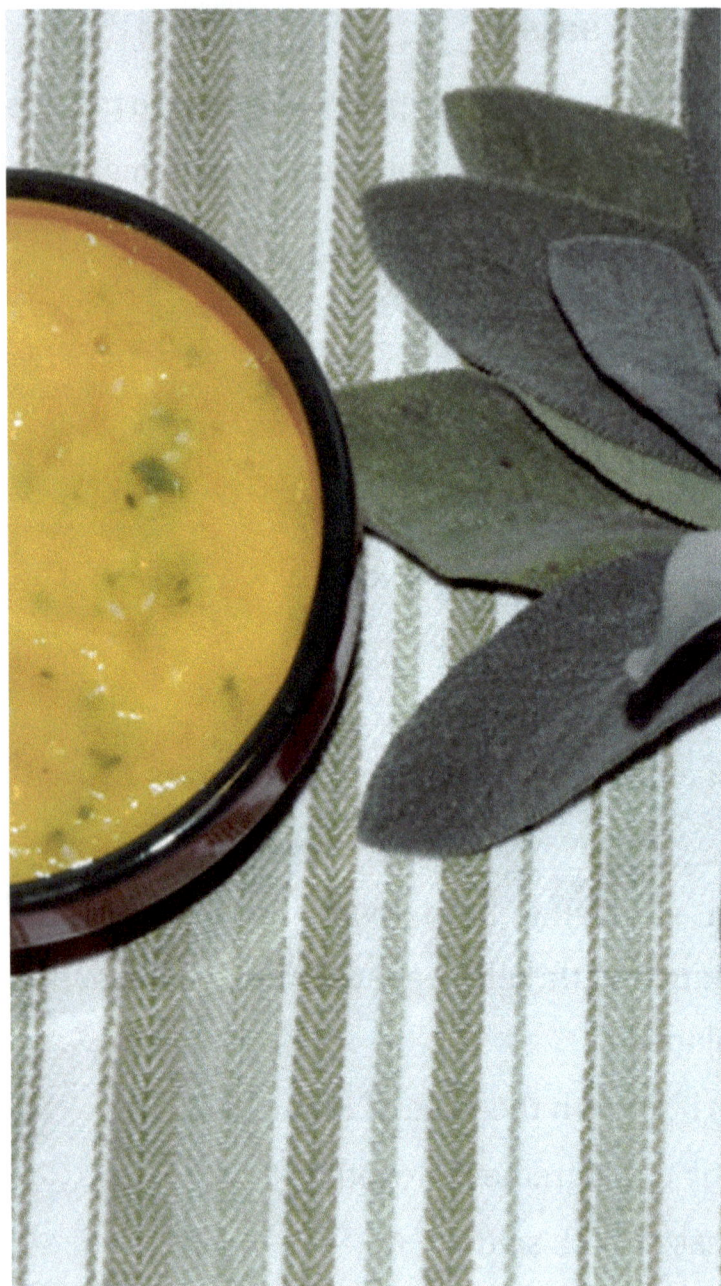

Basil pesto salad dressing

Ingredients

- 4 ounces of chopped romaine lettuce
- ½ cup of fresh basil leaves
- Freshly ground pepper
- 4 ounces of fresh spring greens
- 1 clove garlic
- ¼ teaspoon of salt
- 3 tablespoons of raw pine nuts
- Basil pesto dressing
- ½ cup of extra virgin olive oil
- 2 tablespoons of lemon juice

Directions

- Combine the basil, garlic, and pine nuts in a food blender bowl.
- Pulse until coarsely chopped.
- Drizzle in the olive oil, lemon juice, and salt as the machine is running.
- Season with freshly ground black pepper and blend until smooth.
- Serve and enjoy.

Simple beet arugula and feta salad with balsamic thyme dressing

Ingredients

- ¼ cup of crumbled feta
- 2 tablespoons of pepitas
- Balsamic thyme dressing
- 2 medium red beets
- Handful of arugula, roughly chopped

Directions

- Toast the pepitas over a medium heat until fragrant.
- Transfer to a bowl to cool.
- Prepare and stack the rounds of beets on top of each other and slice them into long, thin matchsticks.
- In a medium-sized serving bowl, combine the beets together with the arugula, crumbled feta, and pepitas.
- Drizzle in enough dressing to coat the salad once tossed.
- Serve and enjoy.

Peach and avocado green salad

Ingredients

- ½ teaspoon of Dijon mustard
- ½ small red onion
- 1 clove garlic, pressed
- ¼ cup of extra virgin olive oil
- 12 ounces of baby arugula
- ¼ teaspoon of ground black pepper
- ¼ cup of freshly squeezed lemon juice
- ⅔ cup of crumbled mild blue cheese
- 2 medium ripe peaches
- 2 medium ripe avocados
- ¾ teaspoon of kosher salt
- ⅔ cup of unsalted sliced almonds

Directions

- Place red onion in a small bowl and cover with water.
- Toast almond in a small skillet over medium-low heat.
- Let cook until the almonds are fragrant, stirring frequently in 5 minutes.

- In a small bowl, whisk extra virgin olive oil, lemon juice, Dijon mustard, garlic, kosher salt, and black pepper.
- Drizzle half of the dressing over the greens, toss.
- Drain the red onion, scatter over the arugula.
- Top with the peaches, avocados, almonds and cheese.
- Serve and enjoy.

Roasted delicata squash, pomegranate, and arugula salad

The roasted delicate squash is a vibrant salad featuring pepitas, feta tossed in a natural balsamic vinaigrette; a perfect choice of Mediterranean Sea diet.

Ingredients

- 1 teaspoon of Dijon mustard
- 2 medium delicata squash
- 2 teaspoons of maple syrup
- 1 ½ tablespoons of balsamic vinegar
- 4 tablespoon of extra virgin olive oil
- Freshly ground black pepper
- Pinch of fine salt
- ¼ teaspoon of fine salt
- 5 ounces of arugula
- Arils from 1 pomegranate
- ⅓ cup of raw pepitas
- 4 ounces of crumbled feta cheese

Directions

- Preheat your oven ready to 425°F.

- Drizzle the squash with a tablespoon of olive oil and sprinkle with salt.
- Bake for 35 minutes in the preheated oven, or until the squash golden, flipping halfway.
- Toast the pepitas in a medium skillet over medium-low heat, stirring frequently, until fragrant in 5 minutes. Remove.
- In a small bowl, whisk together the olive oil with balsamic vinegar, maple syrup, Dijon mustard, and salt.
- Season with black pepper.
- Combine the arugula, pomegranate, pepitas, crumbled feta, and squash in a large serving bowl.
- Drizzle in the dressing and toss to combine.
- Serve and enjoy.

Ginger salad dressing

The ginger salad dressing has a striking flavor drawn from the ginger balanced with sweetness infused with the maple syrup making it a tasty Mediterranean Sea diet recipe.

Ingredients

- ½ cup extra-virgin olive oil
- 2 teaspoons of finely grated fresh ginger
- ½ teaspoon of fine sea salt
- 2 tablespoons of apple cider vinegar
- 20 twists of freshly ground black pepper
- 2 tablespoons of Dijon mustard
- 1 tablespoon of maple syrup

Directions

- In a small mixing bowl, whisk all of the ingredients listed until completely blended.
- Taste the seasoning, and adjust accordingly.
- Serve and enjoy.
- Any leftovers can be kept refrigerated until consumed.

Favorite green salad with apples, cranberries, and pepitas

All the healthy greens you are seeking for are in this Mediterranean Sea diet green salad recipe. It features apples, pepitas, and cranberries.

Ingredients

- 1 teaspoon of Dijon mustard
- 5 ounces of spring greens salad blend
- 1 ½ tablespoons of apple cider vinegar
- 1 ½ teaspoons of honey
- ¼ teaspoon of fine sea salt
- 1 large apple
- ⅓ cup of dried cranberries
- ¼ cup of pepitas
- Freshly ground black pepper
- 2 ounces of chilled goat cheese
- ¼ cup of extra virgin olive oil

Directions

- Toast the pepitas over medium heat in a medium-sized skillet, stirring frequently, until golden on the edges.

- Transfer the pepitas to a small bowl to cool.
- In a small dish, whisk together the olive oil, honey, vinegar, mustard, and salt until well blended.
- Season to taste with pepper.
- Place the greens in a large serving bowl.
- Top with sliced apple, dried cranberries, and toasted pepitas.
- Crumble the goat cheese over the salad.
- Drizzle with enough dressing to lightly coat the leaves once tossed.
- Serve and enjoy.

Roasted beets and labneh

Do you want to boost blood supply in the body? If yes, roasted beets is the best Mediterranean Sea diet recipe you can count on to achieve that; served with avocado and herbs.

Ingredients

- 2 cups of fresh basil leaves
- 4 bunches of beets
- 2 tablespoons of red wine vinegar
- ½ teaspoon of red pepper flakes
- ¼ cup of extra virgin olive oil
- 1 teaspoon of red pepper flakes
- Salt and freshly ground black pepper
- 2 cups of labneh
- 1 clove garlic
- 1 teaspoon of kosher salt
- 3 tablespoons of basil vinaigrette
- 2 ripe avocados
- Fresh mint leaves
- Fresh dill leaves
- 3 shallots, roughly chopped

Directions

- Preheat the oven to 425°F.
- Line a large baking sheet with parchment paper.
- Toss wedges of beets with shallots in olive oil.
- Season with the red pepper flakes, salt and pepper.
- Transfer the seasoned beets and shallots to the prepared baking sheet
- Let roast for 50 minutes, until fork tender.
- Remove, let cool to room temperature.
- Combine the shallot together with basil, red wine vinegar, garlic, red pepper flakes, olive oil, and salt in a blender.
- Let blend until very smooth.
- Season with salt and pepper.
- Spread the labneh on a large platter
- Dollop with basil vinaigrette, scatter with the beets and avocado wedges.
- Then, sprinkle with fresh mint leaves, dill, and flaky salt
- Serve and enjoy.

Honey mustard Brussels sprout slaw

The Brussels sprouts are neatly shredded and tossed with natural tangy honey mustard, finally dressed with almonds and dried cherries. It is a perfect choice of Mediterranean Sea diet for vegans.

Ingredients

- 1 tablespoon of Dijon mustard
- 1 pound of Brussels sprouts
- 1 tablespoon of honey
- ⅓ cup of slivered almonds
- ⅓ cup of tart dried cherries
- 1 garlic clove, pressed
- ¼ teaspoon of fine sea salt
- ⅓ cup of shredded Parmesan cheese
- ¼ cup of extra virgin olive oil
- 2 tablespoons of apple cider vinegar

Directions

- Whisk together the olive oil with vinegar, honey, mustard, and garlic until blended.

- Toss the shredded sprouts in a medium serving bowl with the almonds, chopped dried fruit, Parmesan, and dressing.
- Taste, and adjust accordingly.
- Serve and enjoy immediately.

Layered panzanella salad

Ingredients

- 2 mini cucumbers
- 4 ounces of ciabatta
- 8 ounces of fresh mozzarella
- 2 tablespoons of extra virgin olive oil
- ⅓ cup of roughly chopped fresh basil
- 1 pound of additional tomatoes
- 1 teaspoon fine sea salt
- 3 tablespoons red wine vinegar
- ½ teaspoon dried oregano
- 1 large clove garlic
- 2 tablespoons of thinly sliced Kalamata olives
- Freshly ground black pepper
- ½ small red onion, thinly sliced
- 1 pound of cherry or grape tomatoes

Directions

- Preheat the oven to 425°F.
- Slice the bread and place on the baking sheet.
- Drizzle the cubes with the olive oil and sprinkle with salt, and toss until thoroughly combined.

- Bake until deeply golden 10 minutes.
- In a bowl, combine the olive oil together with the vinegar, oregano, garlic, salt, and black pepper. Whisk to combine.
- Add slice and add onion, or stir into the dressing.
- Refrigerate in the meantime.
- Transfer the prepared tomatoes to a large serving platter.
- Nestle half of the croutons in between the tomatoes, and distribute the rest on top.
- Place the cucumber rounds with the mozzarella all over the salad.
- Sprinkle the basil, olives on top, black pepper and dried oregano on top.
- Serve and enjoy.

Watermelon salad with herbed yogurt sauce

Ingredients

- 1 cup of Greek yogurt
- 2 mini cucumbers
- 1 teaspoon of honey
- Pinch of fine sea salt
- ½ cup of thinly sliced shallot
- 3 tablespoons of sherry vinegar
- ¼ teaspoon of fine sea salt
- 2 tablespoons of extra virgin olive oil
- Small handful fresh mint and basil leaves
- 3 pounds of ripe seedless watermelon
- Flaky sea salt
- Freshly ground black pepper

Directions

- Start by combining the sliced shallot, vinegar, and ¼ teaspoon salt in a small bowl.
- Toss to combine, and refrigerate to pickle.

- Then, in a food processor, combine the yogurt together with the fresh herbs, olive oil, honey, and a pinch of salt.
- Blend until the herbs are broken into tiny pieces and the sauce is pale green.
- Swirl the yogurt sauce over the base of the serving platter.
- Then, scatter the cubed watermelon on top with the cucumber.
- Organize the pickled shallot on top, and spoon the leftover vinegar over the salad.
- Drizzle 2 tablespoons olive oil on top.
- Sprinkle generously with fresh herbs.
- Season with salt and pepper.
- Serve and enjoy chilled.

Mediterranean raw squash pasta salad

This is an incredible couscous salad with a bold raw squash flavors. A typical Mediterranean summer dish delicious enough to keep you hooked on to eating continuously.

Ingredients

- 1 medium zucchini
- ⅓ cup of pitted and thinly sliced Kalamata olives
- 1 ⅓ cup of whole wheat Israeli couscous
- ⅓ cup of pine nuts
- 1 small yellow squash
- ⅓ cup of extra virgin olive oil
- 1 pint of grape tomatoes, quartered
- 4 tablespoons of lemon juice
- ⅓ cup of chopped fresh basil
- 1 large shallot, finely chopped
- 2 cloves garlic, pressed or minced
- 4 ounces of feta cheese
- ½ teaspoon of fine sea salt, to taste
- Freshly ground black pepper

- 1 can of chickpeas, rinsed and drained

Directions

- Cook the couscous according to package directions.
- Drain off any excess water.
- Then toast the pine nut over medium-low heat until turning lightly golden on the sides.
- Transfer to a bowl to cool.
- Whisk together the olive oil with lemon juice, shallot, garlic, salt and many twists of black pepper to combined.
- Add the couscous to the bowl, toss to coat with the dressing.
- Top the couscous with the toasted pine nuts, feta, olives, chickpeas, tomatoes, zucchini, and squash, and basil. Stir to combine.
- Season with salt and pepper to taste.
- Serve and enjoy chilled.

Blood orange and avocado salad

A combination of oranges and avocado is a nutritional blast for brightening yup one's winter days. It is packed with seasonal flavors to tease your taste buds.

Ingredients

- ¼ cup of fresh cilantro leaves
- Flaky sea salt
- ¼ small red onion
- 4 blood oranges
- 1 teaspoon of nigella seed, black sesame seeds
- 2 tablespoons of extra virgin olive oil
- 1 large ripe avocado, thinly sliced
- 2 tablespoons of fresh lime juice

Directions

- Soak the onions for 20 minutes or so in iced water to crisp and softens their flavor intensity.
- On a large serving plate, layer the orange and avocado slices.
- Drain the onion and tuck pieces in between and on top of the orange and avocado.

- Drizzle the salad with the lime juice.
- Sprinkle with salt.
- Sprinkle the seeds and cilantro on top.
- Drizzle with olive oil all over it.
- Serve and enjoy.

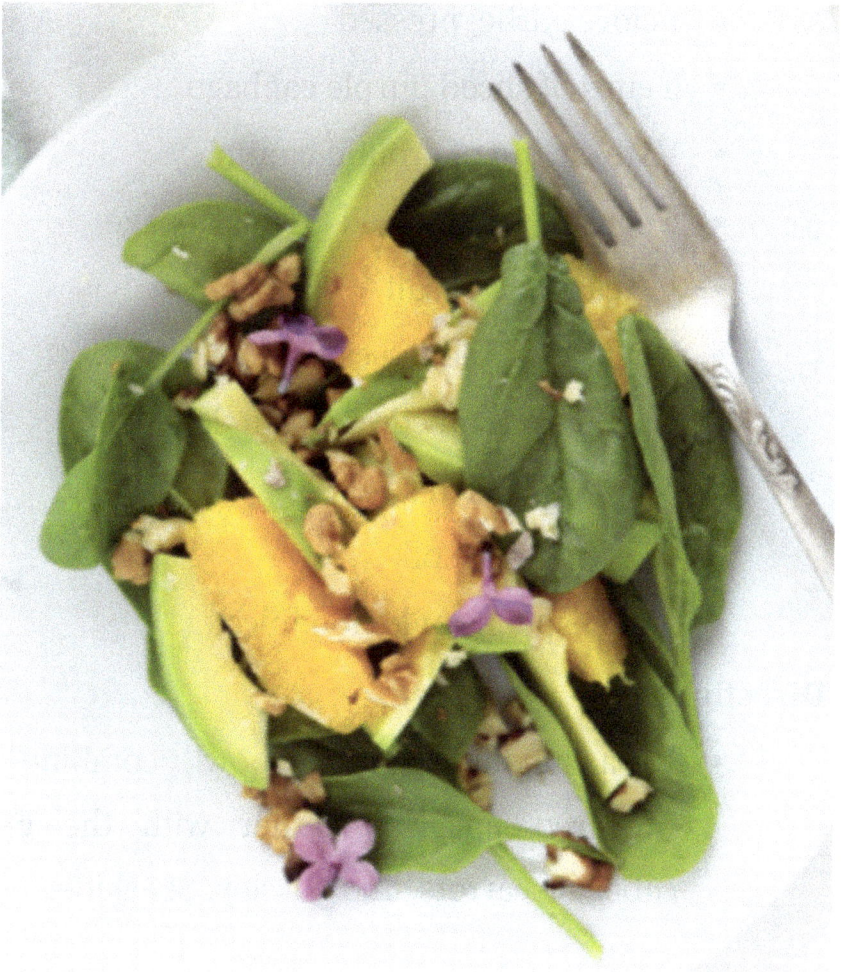

Simple seedy slaw

The simple seedy slaw utilizes a simple lemon dressing to spike up the taste and flavor toasted with pumpkin seeds and sunflower. It is gluten free perfect for a vegan and Mediterranean Sea diet.

Ingredients

- 1 clove garlic, pressed
- 2 cups of sliced purple cabbage
- ½ teaspoon of ground cumin
- 2 cups of finely sliced green cabbage
- ½ teaspoon of salt
- 2 cups of shredded carrots
- ¼ cup of chopped fresh parsley
- ¾ cup of mixed seeds
- ¼ cup of olive oil
- 3 tablespoons of lemon juice

Directions

- In a medium serving bowl, combine the prepared purple together with the green cabbage, carrots, and parsley. Set aside.

- Toast seeds over medium heat, stirring frequently, until the seeds are fragrant.
- Pour the toasted seeds into the mixing bowl and toss to combine.
- In a small bowl, combine the olive oil together with 2 tablespoons of lemon juice.
- Then, add the garlic with cumin and salt, whisk until blended.
- Drizzle the dressing over the slaw, toss until ingredients are coated in dressing.
- Serve and enjoy.

www.ingramcontent.com/pod-product-compliance
Lightning Source LLC
Chambersburg PA
CBHW050755030426
42336CB00012B/1825